My Dad

Dealing with FTD

My Dad

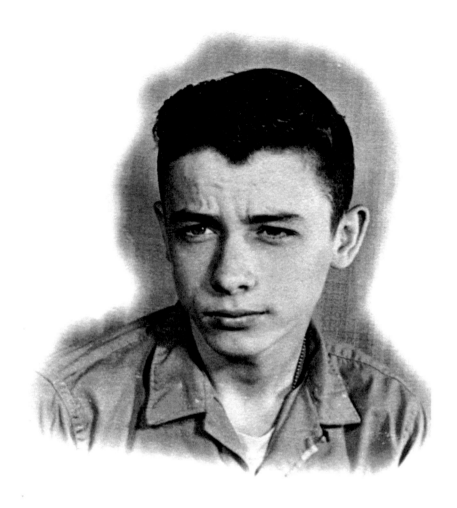

Al Shoberg - High School Senior

In just a few short years, he will meet my mom, get married, get drafted, survive Vietnam, come home, have a family and settle down for the long haul. I was born first, in 1972, then came my brother, and whoops! then came my sister. Our little family has been through a lot, but my dad always made us feel loved and rich. Whether we were camping, vacationing, or simply visiting, we were given everything a kid could need. Maybe it wasn't always what we wanted, but we always had what we needed.

This book outlines the life of my dad, with pictures from before this wretched diagnosis until now. When my dad was diagnosed with FTD, Frontotemporal Degeneration, we had no idea what that was. First we were told it was Pick's Disease. I didn't know what that was either. A friend nodded sagely when I told him my dad had Pick's, but he didn't explain it. My mom was anxious about it. We kids were unsure what to think. When it finally came out as FTD, we were told he had anywhere from 5-8 years to live. We were told that FTD was not Alzheimer's or ALS. It wasn't any other form of dementia, but it would manifest as a type of dementia. It could affect his behavior, meaning he could have a personality change. He might get mean, or he might get euphoric. He might get timid or anxious. It could affect his speech, meaning he might lose the ability to speak. He might repeat what we say or have a stammer. It could affect his executive functioning, meaning he may not be able to dress himself, or feed himself, or do any chores anymore. What it came down to was any differences we see are probably due to the FTD. Not a promising way to watch your father decline. Father's are supposed to be strong, be a girl's hero.

And he was all of that, but now he's the one who needs us to be strong. His FTD affected his speech. He stammers so much that he can hardly get a word out. He repeats what he is told. So when I hug him and say, "Hi, Dad." He hugs me back and says, "Hi, Dad." For now, I can still get him to call me by name, but that will pass as the disease gets worse. It has also affected his behavior. He gets up at night and gets dressed thinking it's time, even at 3am. He is unstable in his motion, but doesn't use a walker or a cane yet. That will also come. He acts like a 5 year old at times, like when he wants to kick out the feet from the walker in front of him. And it also affects his executive functioning. He has a hard time getting dressed sometimes, and he gets confused a lot. But that's now. Let these pictures show you how he was and then maybe you'll know how wretched this bastard disease really is.

Dad, I already miss you. Love you.

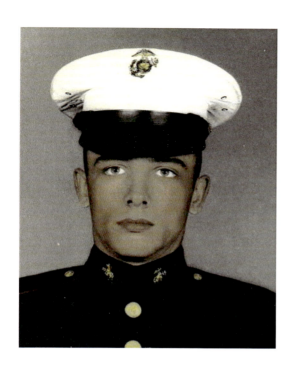

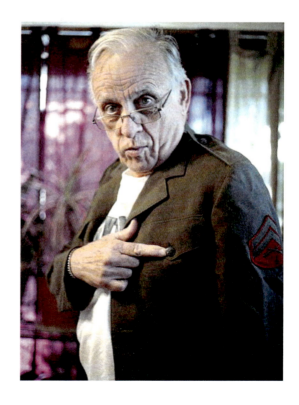

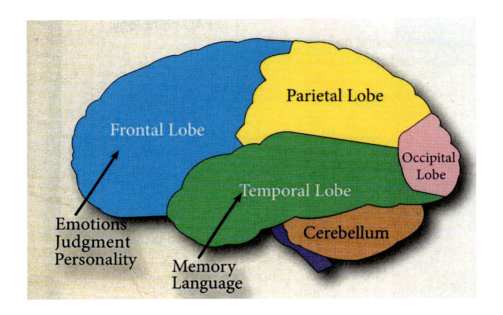

FTD stands for Frontotemporal Dementia. It is also called FTLD, or Frontotemporal Lobe Degeneration, and Pick's Disease. With this disease, both the frontal lobe and the temporal lobe of the brain deteriorate.

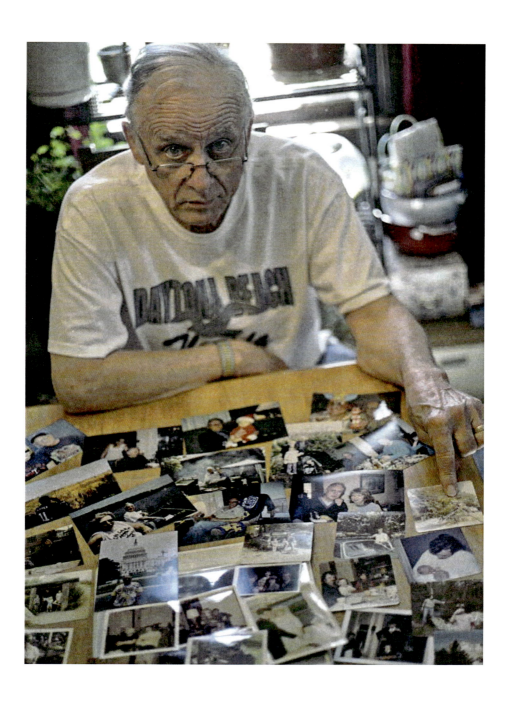

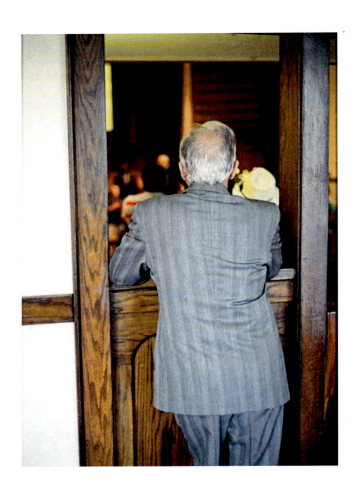

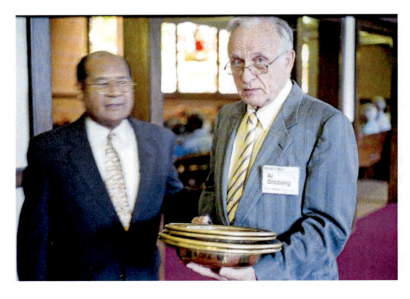

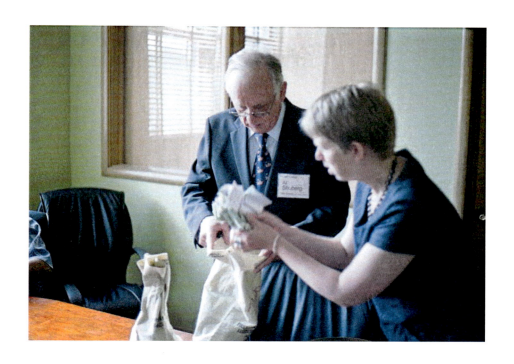

"Al,

    You have been a pillar of the church through your dedicated service as head usher. Quietly, you have lead us by example, teaching us all that we know: service, commitment, dependability, and dedication. Congratulations!"

- Marcus Grice

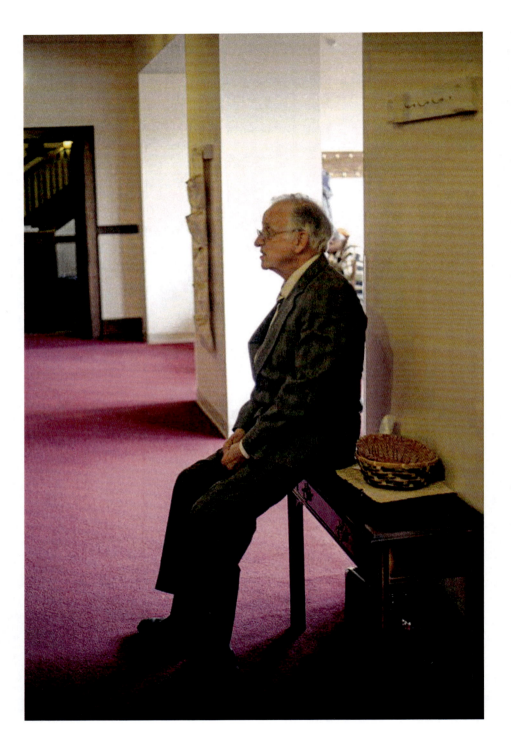

Early symptoms of FTD generally develop in one of three main areas of functioning: language and communication, personality and behavior, or movement and motor skills.

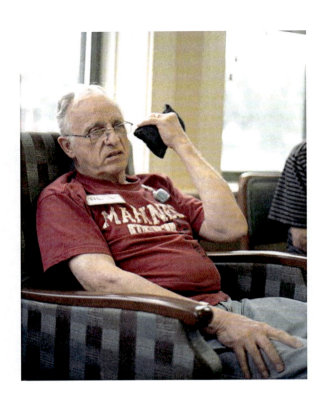

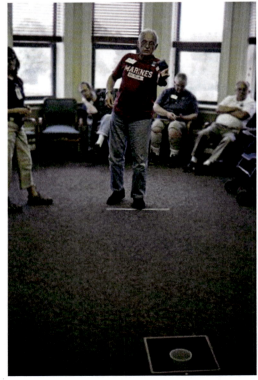

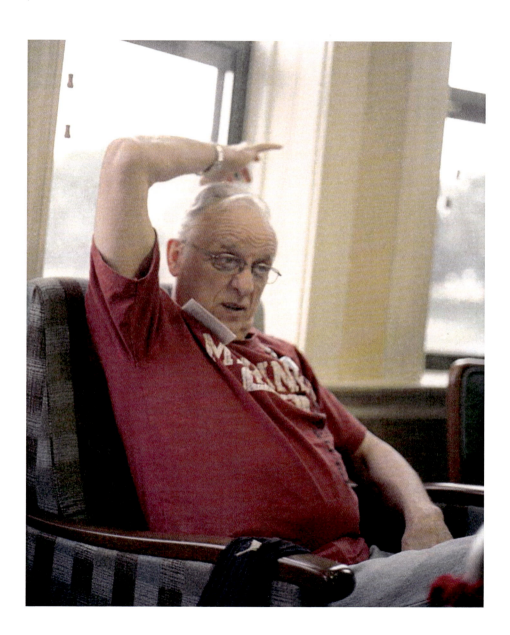

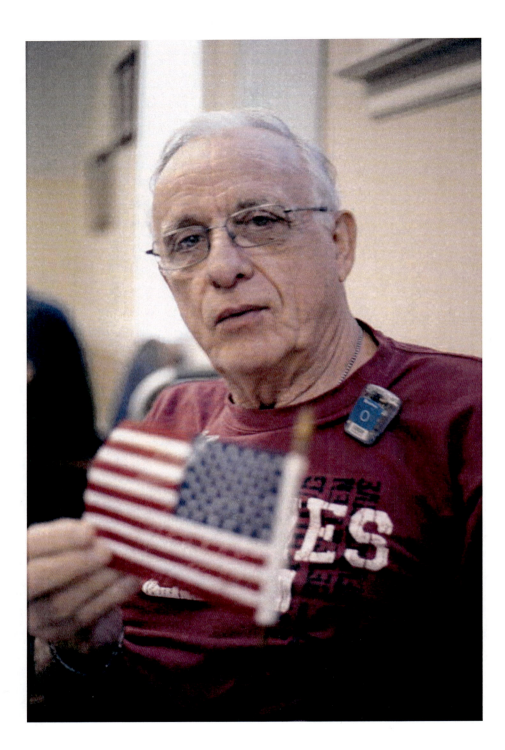

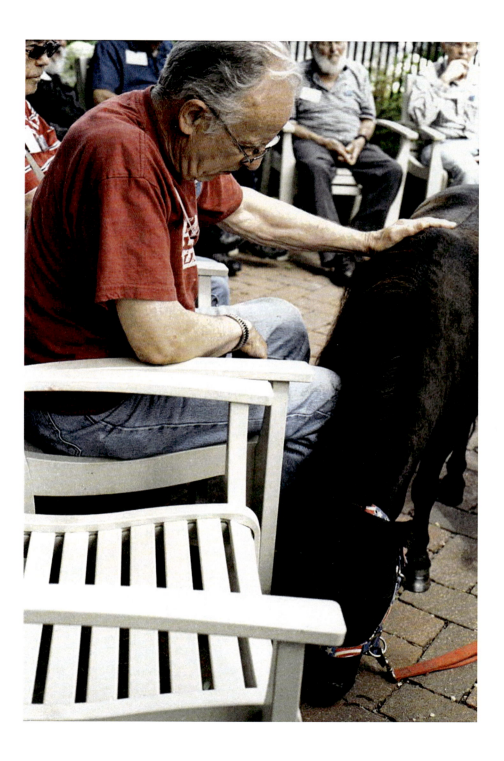

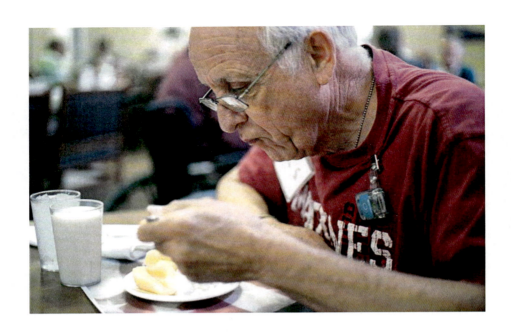

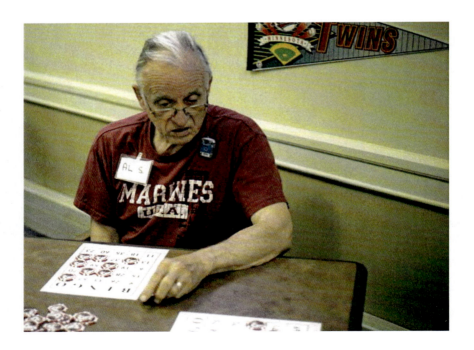

"The Adult Day Center, located in Building 4 on the Minnesota Veterans Home - Minneapolis campus is a Veteran-based community that allows participants to connect with other Veterans in a safe, comfortable environment. The Adult Day Center allows Participants to achieve the highest attainable level of physical, mental and social well-being – with the independence of living at home."

- Taken from the MN VA website

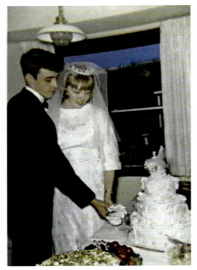

"When I met Al in 1964, he was an 18-year-old high school student who survived a difficult childhood, had lots of brothers, loved to ride his bike as fast as he could, worked several hours a week at a restaurant and was determined to graduate from high school. We dated, fell in love (or lust) and got married August 28, 1965 against his family's wishes because I was 3 years older than he and a dreaded Protestant.

He was drafted into the Marines shortly after we were married and we lived in Oceanside, CA while he trained for Vietnam. During his deployment, I lived with my parents in Burnsville and my Mom, an experienced military wife, helped me through.

Al was always fun loving, funny and talkative. He loved fixing things for anyone who needed help. He also loved (loves) the Vikings. The week after we were married we went camping with the church. He was captivated by the message delivered by the pastor and he decided that he needed God in his life. He became a devout Christian. After we joined Park Avenue Church, he served as an usher and eventually became head usher. He also was a Cub Scout leader and a member of Toast Masters.

We always loved to travel and collected drinking glasses from every state we visited. Travel and camping were two of our favorite things, especially after we had our 3 children. Our plan for retirement was to travel more overseas and expand our horizons."

- Terri Shoberg

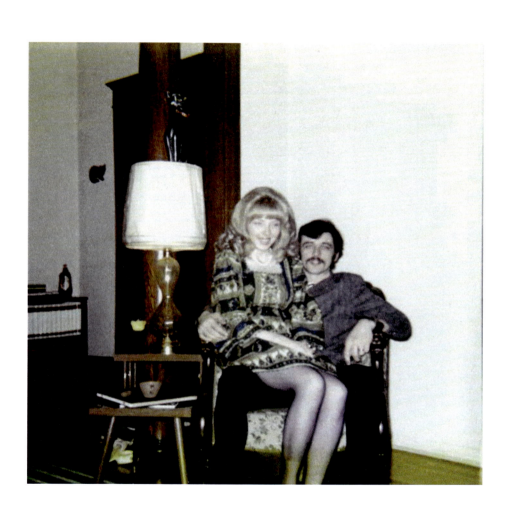

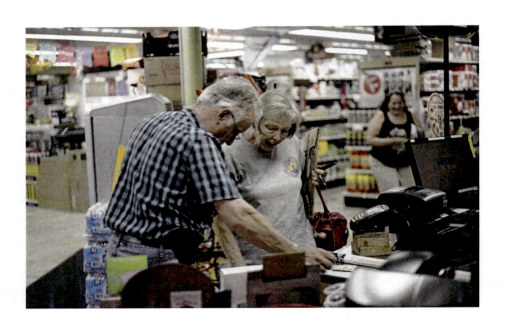

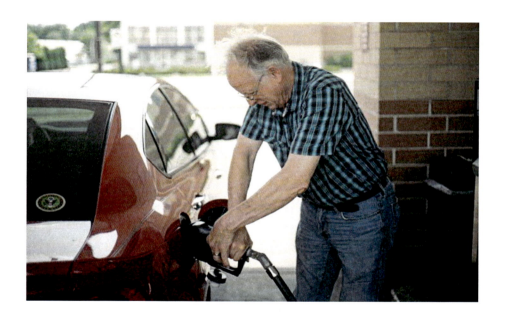

Approximately 50,000 to 70,000 people in the United States are diagnosed with a form of Frontotemporal Degeneration (FTD)

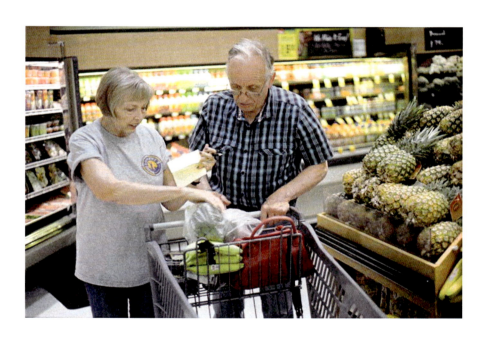

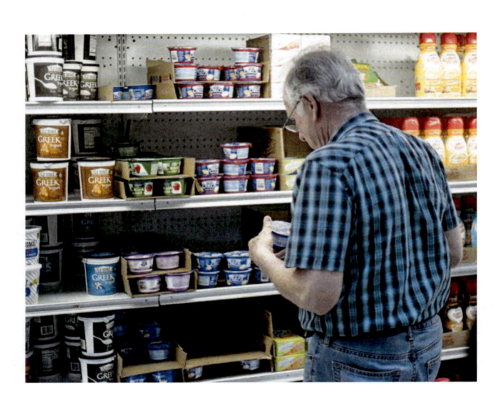

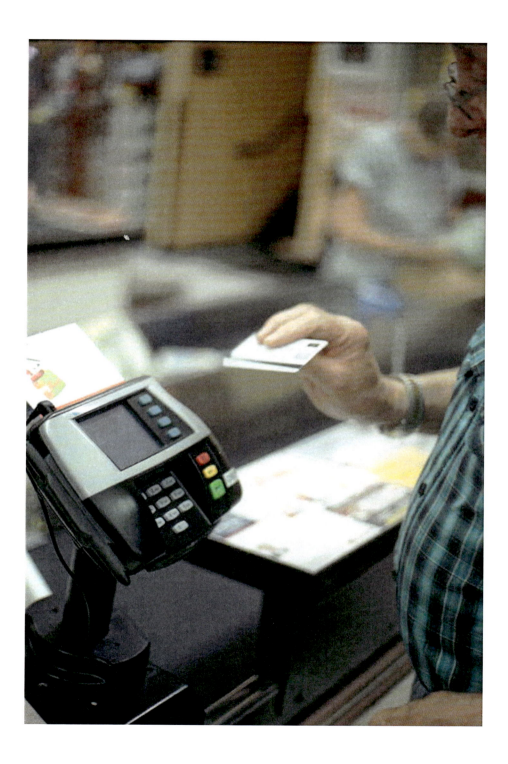

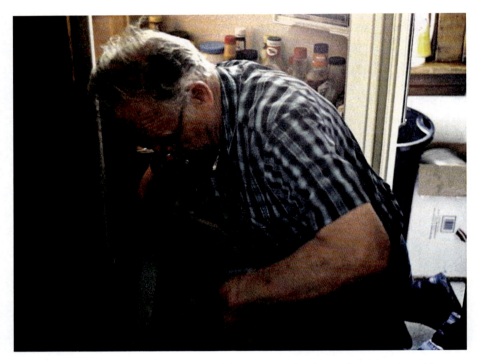

There are no treatments available currently that slow or stop the progression of the disease once it has started.

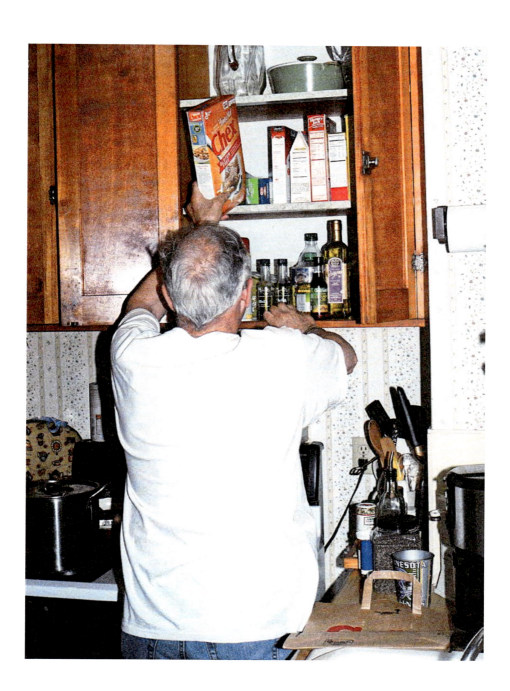

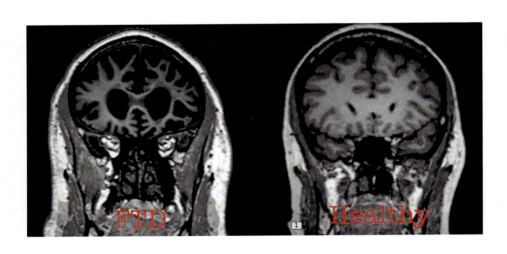

Symptoms of frontotemporal disorders vary from person to person and from one stage of the disease to the next as different parts of the frontal and temporal lobes are affected. In general, changes in the frontal lobe are associated with behavioral symptoms, while changes in the temporal lobe lead to language and emotional disorders.

It is important to understand that people with these disorders cannot control their behaviors and other symptoms.

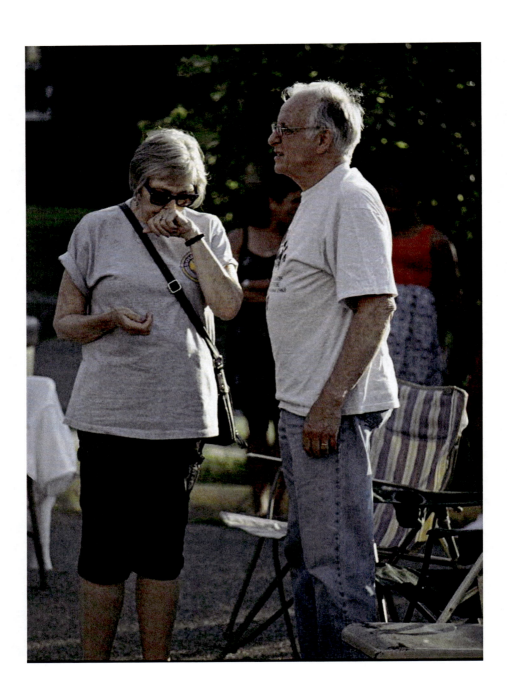

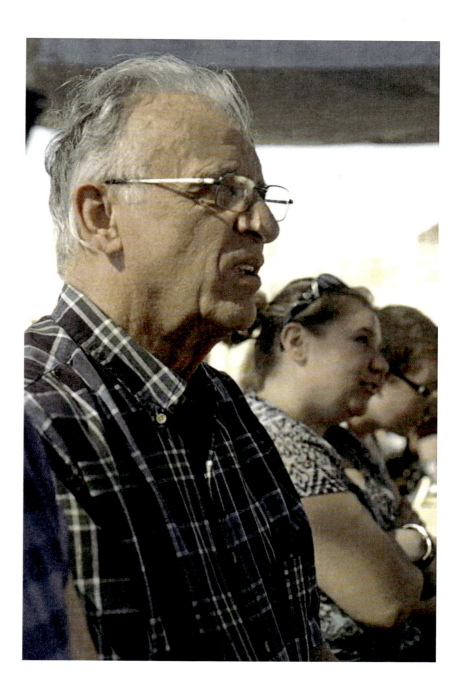

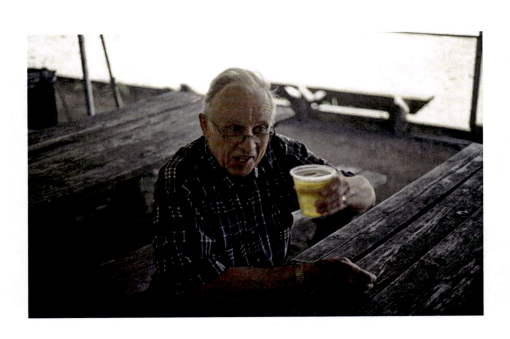

One of my fondest memories of my dad are my birthdays as a child. I remember every year, he would take me, and my brother and sister, to the Picadilly Circus. I got to play games and always had our pictures taken in the picture booth to hang on the kitchen cabinet at home. I always enjoyed my time with my dad at the circus. Then came when I was 12 years old and a little too old to go to the Picadilly Circus, or maybe it was no longer around, but it was a year early for me to get my ears pierced, but dad wanted me to do it. So, at age 12 instead of 13, I got my ears pierced. A special treat for me!!"

- Liz (Shoberg) Borchert

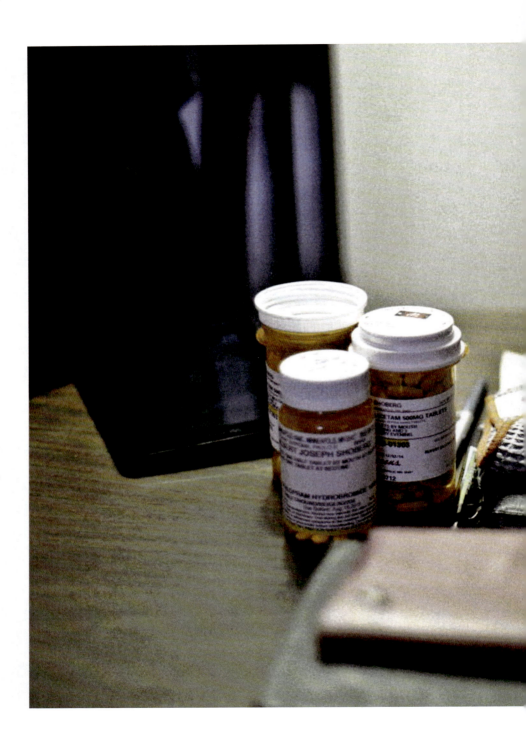

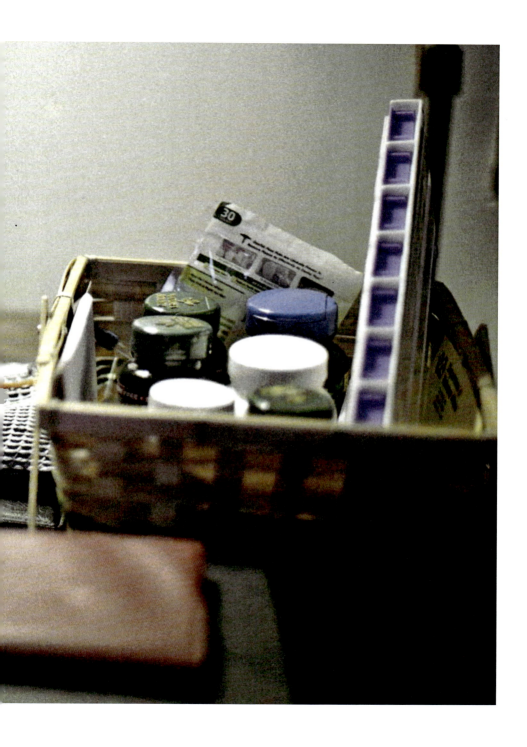

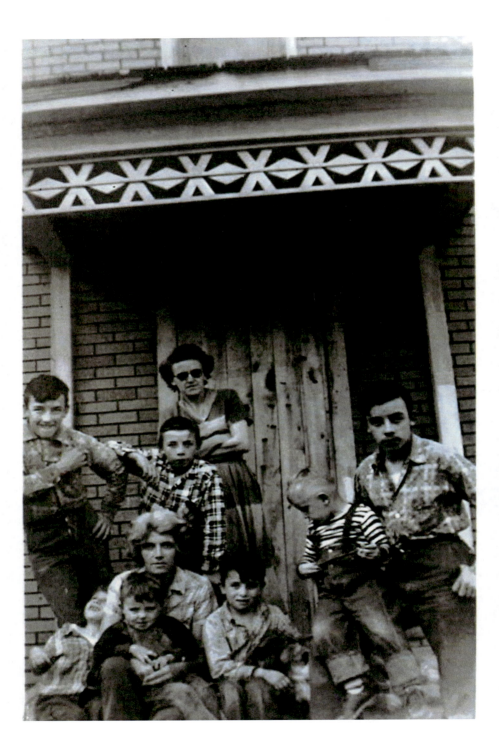

The most effectiveapproach for managing FTD is not linear, but spiral. FTD is progressive and the symptoms you face will change over time.

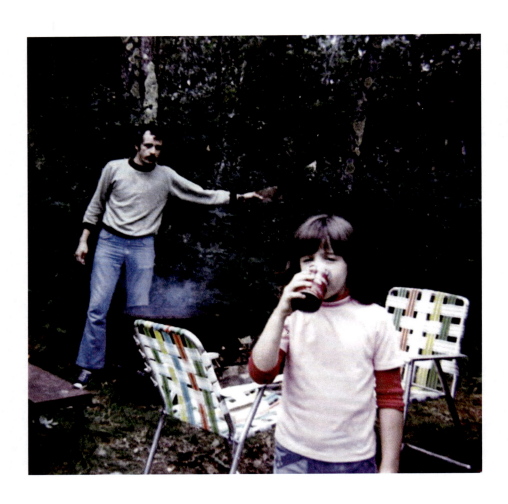

"I first got to know Al in about 1973 when I joined the Koinonia Group that Al and Terri were in. They were great friends at the right time for me. I remember phoning their number from the phone at Bethel Seminary when I attended there in 1974-75. It felt like calling home. From that point came the beginning of thirty-five years of Family Camp at beautiful Star Lake Camp in Cross Lake...

So many things come to memory about Al through all the years of Family Camp. If anyone was arriving late, Al would stay up and keep the camp fire in the Shelter going and wait up for them until they arrived, no matter how late it was. Then he would help set up their tent, screen house, bring his lantern or whatever they needed to get bedded down for what was left of the night. Even when no one was coming late, Al and I would sit up late for endless nights by that fire in the shelter (Al was the official and consummate fire builder!), watching those beautiful coals and frequently eat any left over popcorn he always popped for the Saturday night community pot-luck dinner and campfire event. But, our favorite late night snacks were summer sausage and cheese and crackers.

Umm! NO family camp was complete without as many rounds of horseshoes as we could get in. I am sure the all time win-loss record between us was about 50-50! Then there was the night that seems like a hundred years ago when the summer air was so still and heavy and the lake so calm that it sounded like every fish in the lake was jumping out of the water. So, we said, "Let's go fishing, they should almost jump right into the canoe!" After a couple hours and not one bite OR a fish in the canoe, we had to give up! But the years of wading through the woods to get to Lake Henry to fish with the kids in the early years were somewhat more successful.

But how can we mention Family Camp without remembering the two straight-line, high wind storms (among many others) that came through Shoberg's camp site just three years apart. It was only God's miracle that all walked away without much damage! There were plenty of other "Divine Interventions" connected with getting to and from camp over the years as well.

Another joint effort with Al was frequently helping each other - and frequently other family campers - keep our cars started or running. He or I could be seen crawling under someone's car in the sand to wire up a tailpipe or muffler. The one memorable car repair job was fixing the transmission of the old Dodge Aspen Station Wagon after the family's trip to South Dakota, I believe. We were wrestling that thing around on the work bench in Al's cramped shop in the basement, but we finally got it back to working smoothly! Possibly the last car caper was in August 2008 when Al and I drove to Oregon pulling a car trailer with Abe's hot Buick in tow. We thought we were going home empty, only to find out Abe or a friend had a car that they wanted to have brought back to Minnesota! The only - but real - headache was repeatedly blowing the fuse on the van circuit that the trailer lights were hooked to. It seems like we had to stop every hundred miles to try to fix it, but we finally made it home safe and sound. And the taste of those fresh, Washington cherries we bought from a stand on the way out still lingers in our mouths!"

_ Gil Kahle

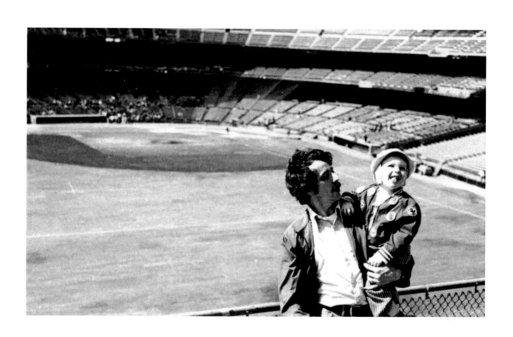

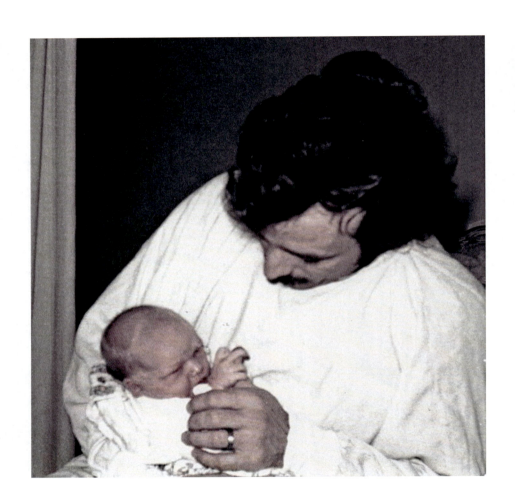

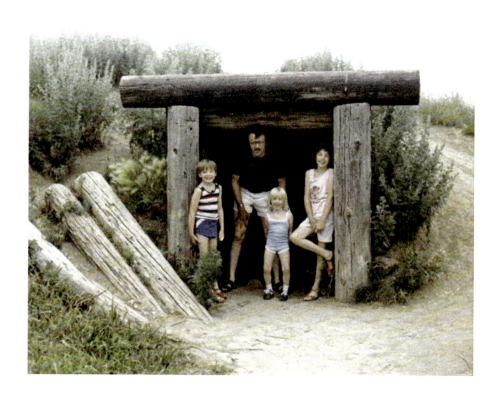

The ultimate cause of FTD is unkown.

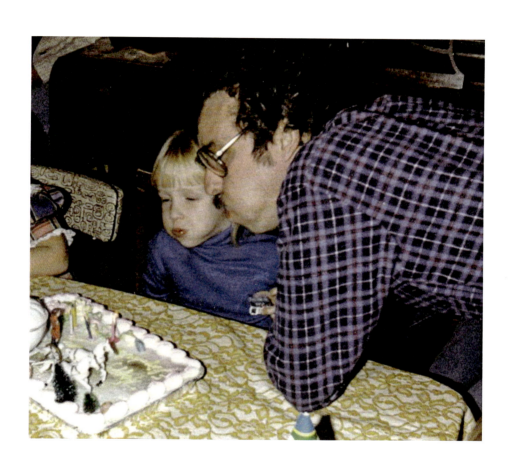

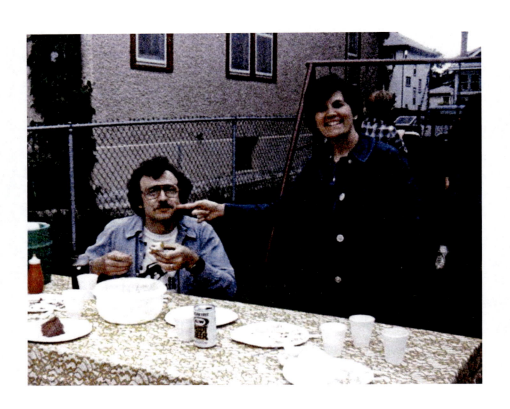

"Many years ago, Al found out that I loved raspberries. He started making me a raspberry pie for my birthday in August and bringing it over so the four of us could eat it. Al's birthday is also in August and I decided I should do something for him for his birthday. Terri told me Al loves banana cream pie and so do I. So I started making a banana cream pie for his birthday. Now every year we both look forward to our pies in August.

When Matt was 7 months old, Gilbert and I were going to my brother's wedding and needed a babysitter. We could not find anyone to care for Matt. At that time, Terri worked evenings and Al stayed home with their kids. Al volunteered to take care of Matt. He was so good with kids, I knew he would not have any problems. As it turned out, Gilbert was sick and couldn't go to the wedding, so I took Matt over to Shoberg's and it was a very relaxing evening."

- Sue Kahle

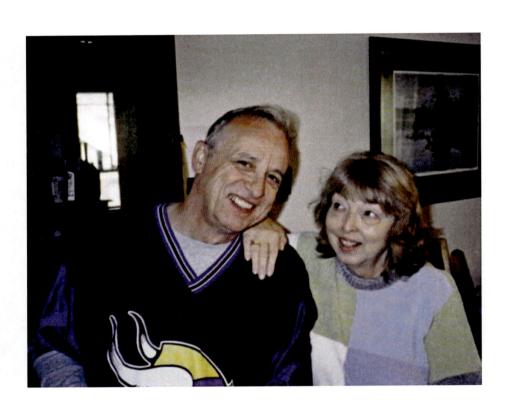

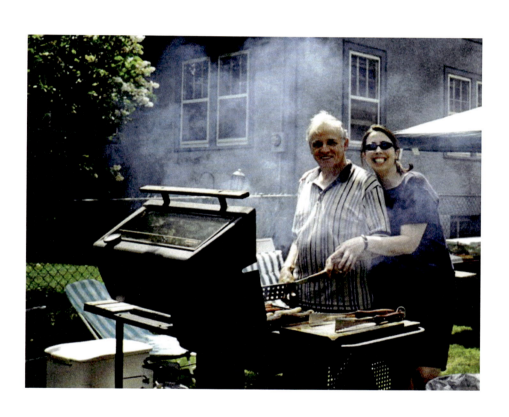

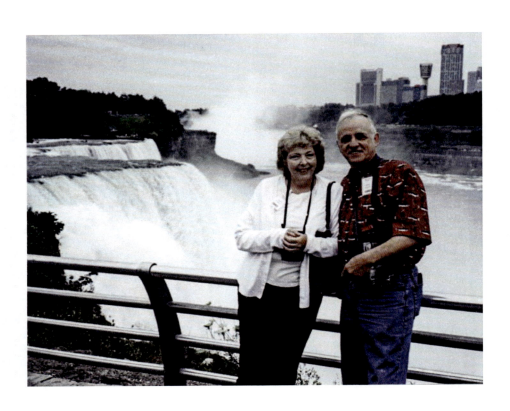

"One of my fondest memories of my father really just involves him and myself hanging out together; just being together and not saying much but knowing everything is ok. This usually revolved around a car, a fast car usually, unless it was his van. One day, eight years ago I was in the middle of restoring the Grand National I bought a year prior. The headliner, the 'ceiling' of the car, was sagging, so I had removed it to get it redone and now was trying to get it back in the car. At the time, I was living in an apartment, so I was at my parents' house doing this work. It was a nice summer day and I didn't think anyone was there. After getting all the trim off, my father came walking down the back walk and asked what I was doing. I told him and he climbed in the car to see what was going on. I was having trouble keeping the headliner up so that I could get the light fixture back on, but my father offered to help. He had a torn rotator cuff so he really only had his left arm to do anything. He laid back, told me to hold on for a second, grabbed his right arm with his left hand and raised it up to postion it so I could get the light put back on. Something about him making that effort to use his otherwise useless arm to hold something for me was pretty cool. He helped me get it all back together and then we went for a cruise. It was nice and I will always remember that."

- Abe Shoberg

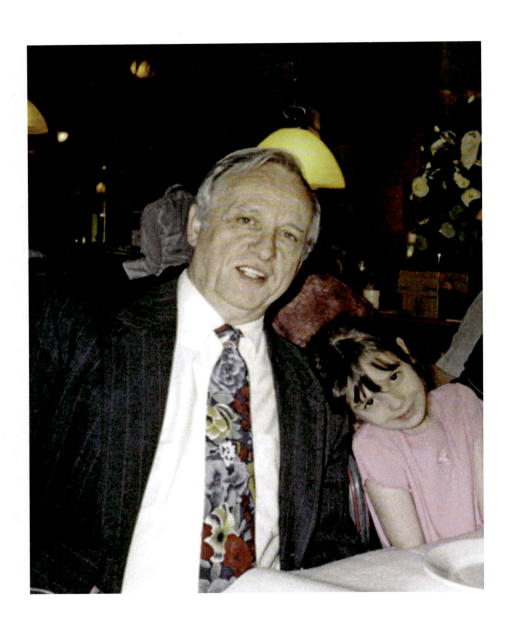

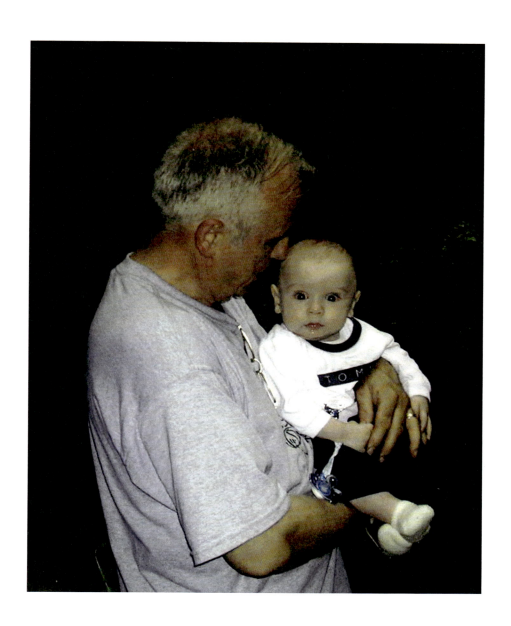

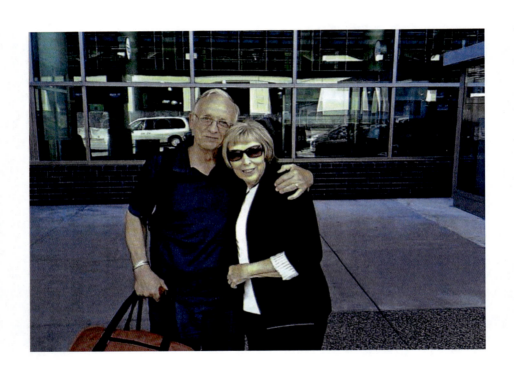

Scientists estimate that FTLD may cause up to 10% of all cases of dementia and may be about as common as Alzheimer's among people younger than 65.

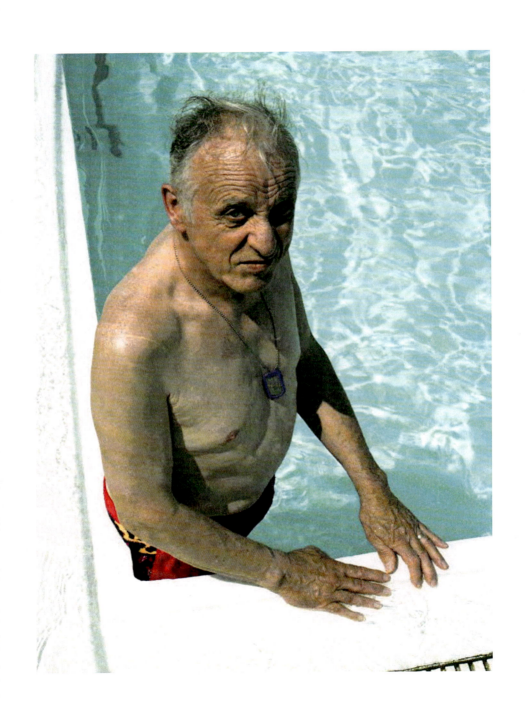

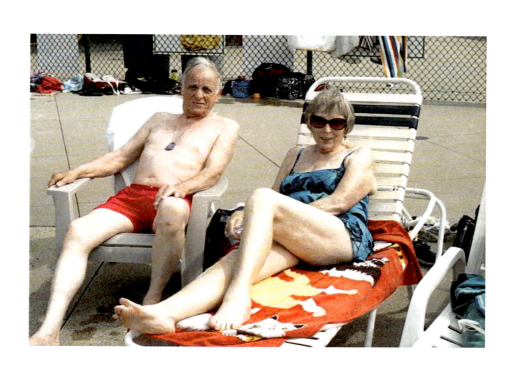

Frontotemporal lobar degeneration (FTLD) is not a single brain disease but rather a family of neurodegenerative diseases, any one of which can cause a frontotemporal disorder.

FTLD can only be definitively identified after death, by brain autopsy.

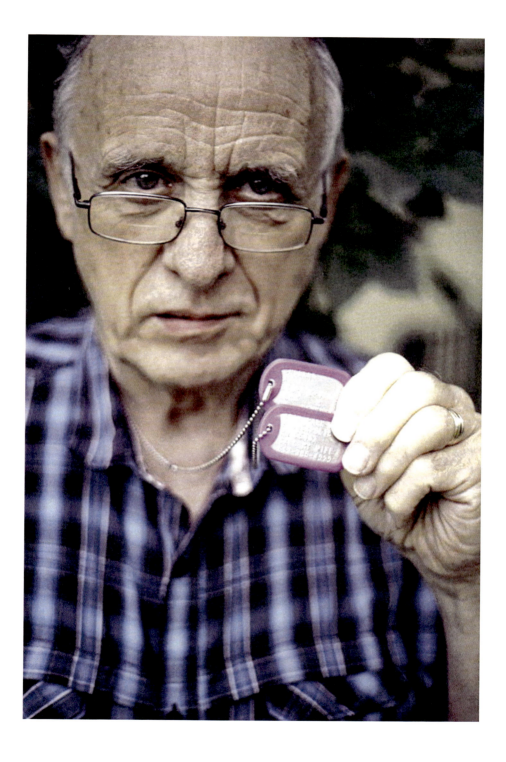

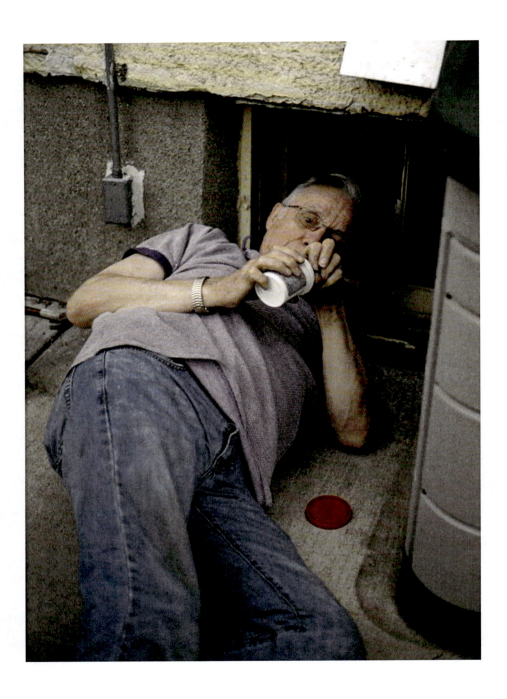

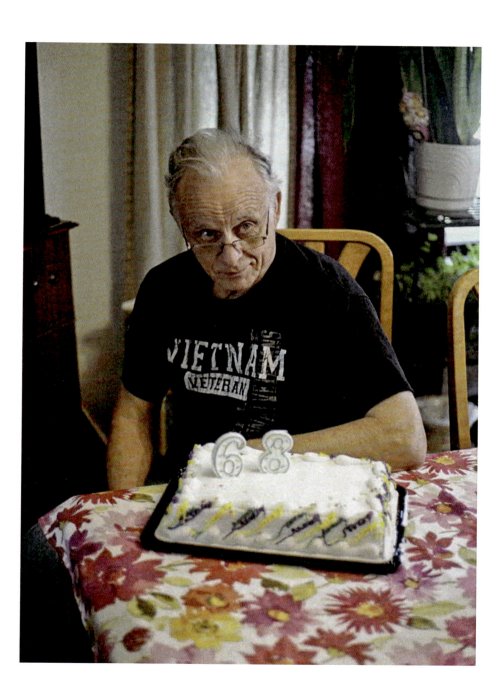

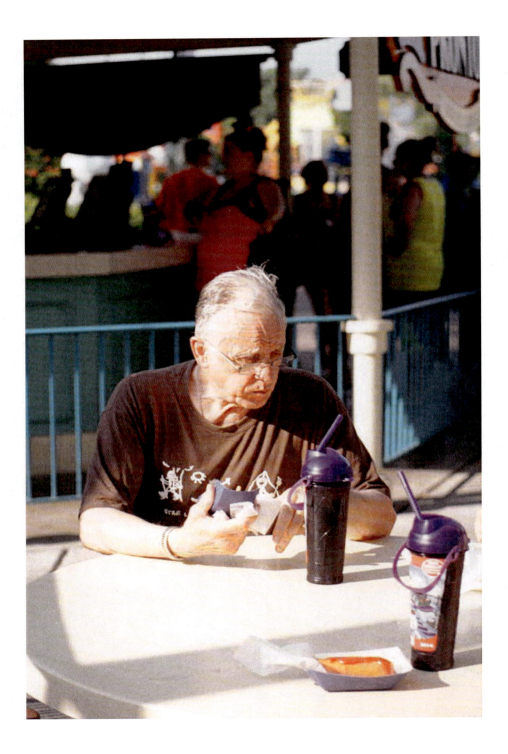

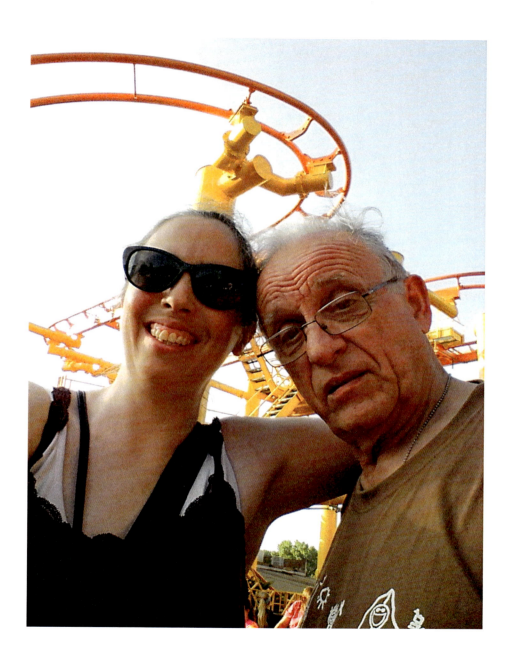

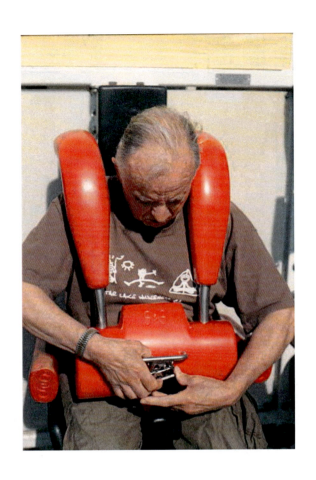

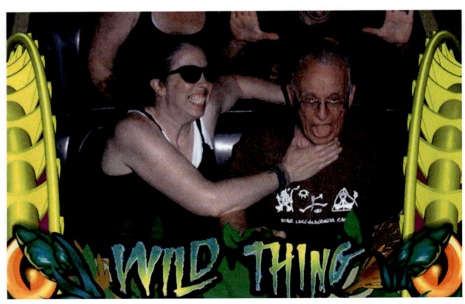

One of the many memories I have of my dad, I have to acknowledge Valleyfair. Since I can remember as a child, he took us to Valleyfair every year in August for his birthday. The trip was his birthday present to himself. He loved the roller coasters and the water rides. He took us on the rides we wanted to go on, but still made it a point, when we were tall enough, to take us on the roller coasters. I remember the High Roller and nearly flying out of the seat because I was just tall enough to ride it, and hating it. I also hated that I was too tall for the kid rides that I still liked. Now of course, we take him, and we all do the roller coasters. This year was yours, Dad. Hope you had fun!

- Jen (Shoberg) Steffen

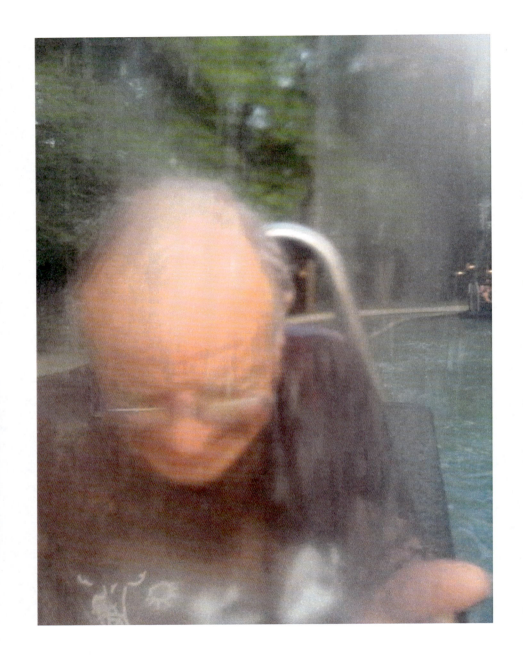

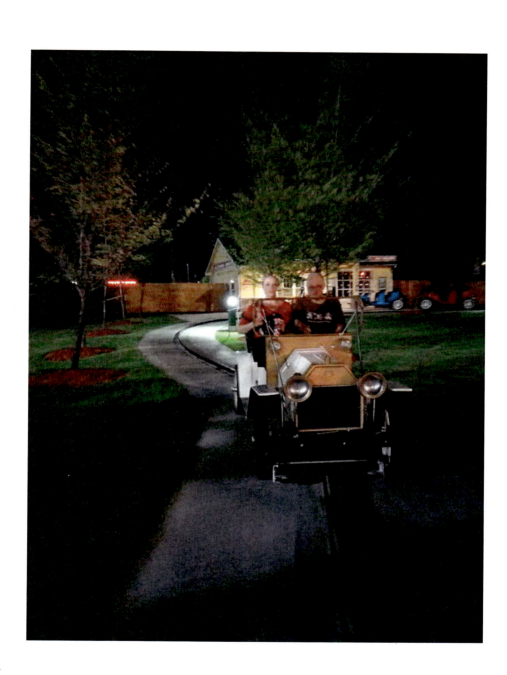

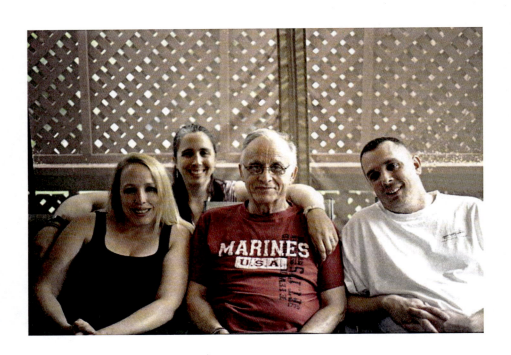

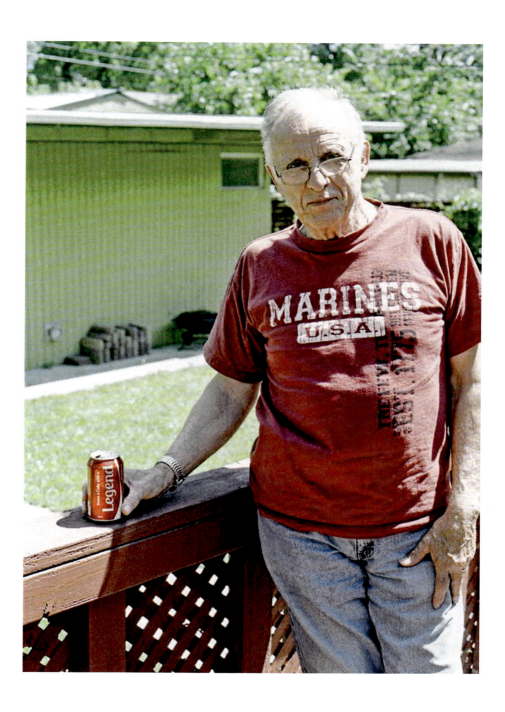

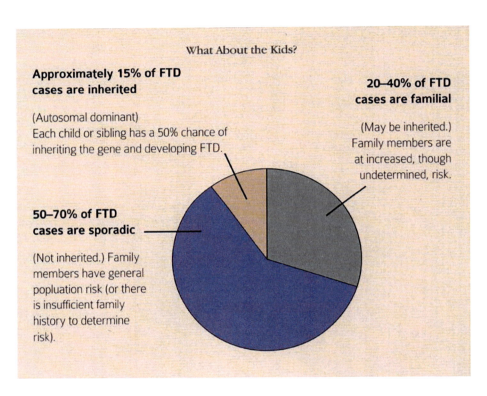

What About the Kids?

Approximately 15% of FTD cases are inherited

(Autosomal dominant)
Each child or sibling has a 50% chance of inheriting the gene and developing FTD.

20–40% of FTD cases are familial

(May be inherited.)
Family members are at increased, though undetermined, risk.

50–70% of FTD cases are sporadic

(Not inherited.) Family members have general popluation risk (or there is insufficient family history to determine risk).

Approximately 40% of individuals with FTD have a family history that indicates at least one other relative who also has or had a neurodegenerative disease.

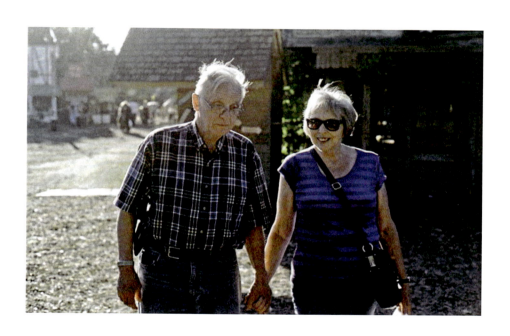

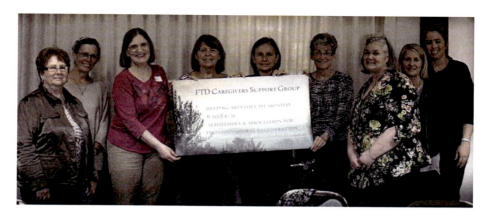

Bibliography

Ruth, Paul. "How FTD Hides." *The Huffington Post*. New York, 22 8 2013.
	E-Newspaper. <www.huffingtonpost.com/paul-ruth/frontotemporal-
	dementia_b_3770455.html>.

The Association for Frontotemporal Degeneration. *The Doctor Thinks
	It's FTD. Now What?* Brochure. Radnor: The Association for
	Frontotemporal Degeneration, 2013. Print.

—. *What About the Kids?* Brochure. Radnor: The Association for
	Frontotemporal Degeneration, 2012. Print.

The Trustees of the University of Pennsylvania. *Understanding the Genetics
	of FTD*. Brochure. Pennsylvania: Penn Medicine, 2012. Print.
	<pennmedicine.org>.

U.S. Department of Health and Human Services. *Frontotemporal Disorders*.
	Brochure. Silver Spring: National Institute of Health, 2010. Print.

This book has come together through the support of family and friends. A few of them wish to remain annonymous, but those who have allowed me, I want to thank by name. They are listed only in alphabetical order.

Jerome Belton
Diane Chynewith
Bill Cottman
Stan Cyr
Tim Fahs
Sherri Hildebrandt
Terri Shoberg
Diana Simplair
Linda Tate

Thank you so much. This would never have come to fruition without your help.

Notes: